DEATH *my* DIARY

A Guided Journal
for Mortals

ANITA HANNIG

sourcebooks

Published by Sourcebooks
P.O. Box 4410, Naperville, Illinois 60567–4410
(630) 961-3900
sourcebooks.com

Printed and bound in the United States of America.
VP 10 9 8 7 6 5 4 3 2 1

Today I,

_____,

am getting curious about my mortality.

Date: ___ / ___ / ___

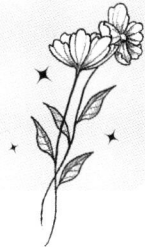

Make your life joyful
by putting aside
all your anxiety
about keeping it.

Seneca, Moral Epistles

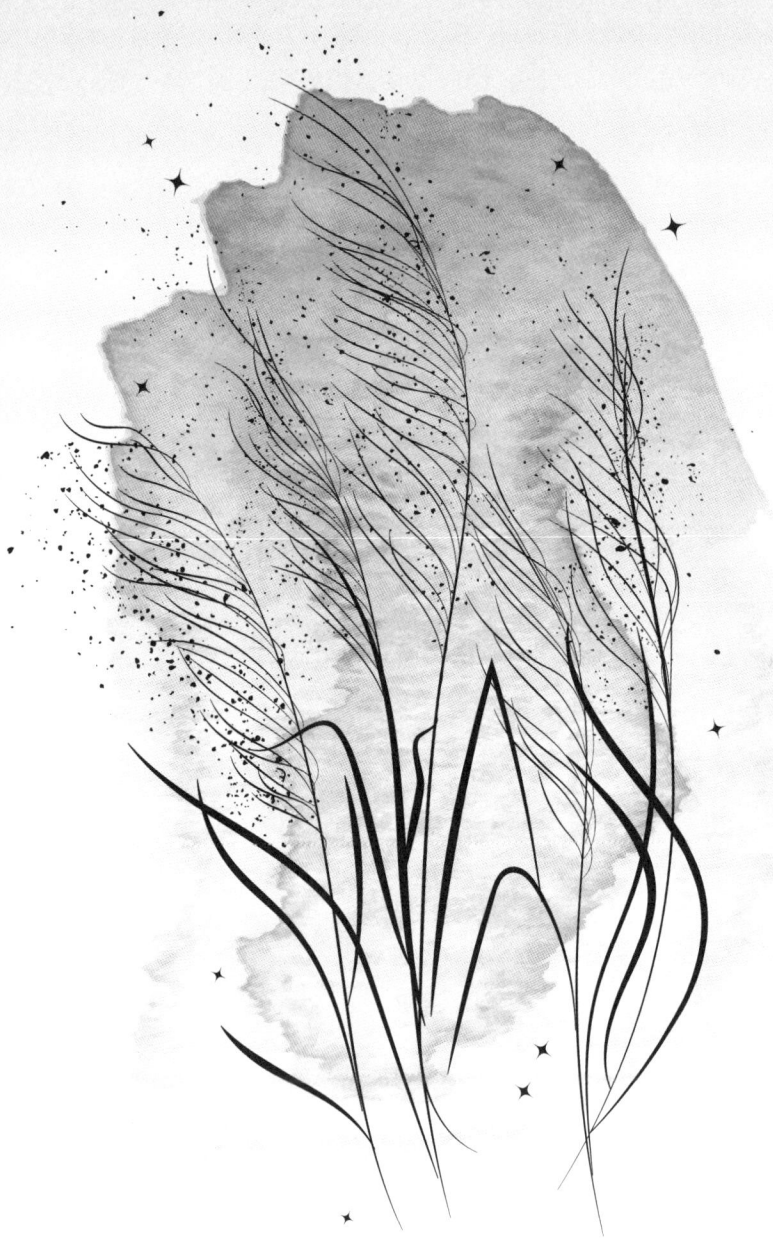

DEAR JOURNALER,

Contemplating death is scary. Most of us prefer not to dwell on the fact that our time here is limited. It feels unnerving to admit that this will all end. Though we spend our entire existence in the shadow of mortality, we like to imagine that we will live forever.

And yet, death is an integral and important part of life. Thousands of years ago, the Roman philosopher Seneca counseled readers not only to accept death but to study it— even to rehearse for it. Seneca believed that nothing was worth having unless you were prepared to let it go.

This journal is your rehearsal. It draws from my years of teaching a class on death and dying to college students, and from my long-term research with patients seeking medical aid in dying. Rather than shield you from your mortality, this journal will give you the space and tools to explore your own relationship with it.

Doing this work isn't easy; it requires a great deal of courage, commitment, and reflection. But trust me, it is worth it. Because nothing brings you more immediately into the present than the realization that life is finite.

What if you used this time—right now—to no longer simply ignore or fear death but to prepare and equip yourself for it?

The benefits of reflecting on your mortality in this structured way are incalculable. Not only will death appear much less spooky and daunting; you might also gain a renewed appreciation for life.

Let's dive deep together.

Anita

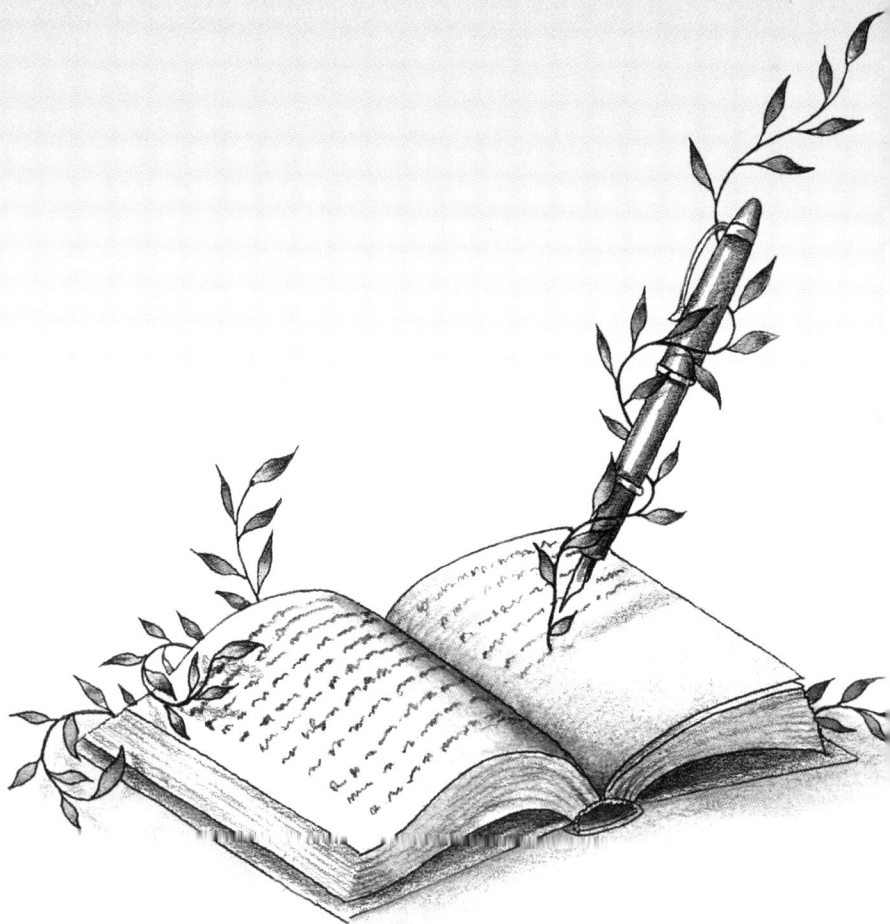

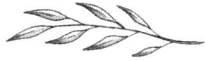

GETTING STARTED

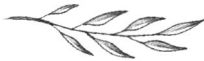

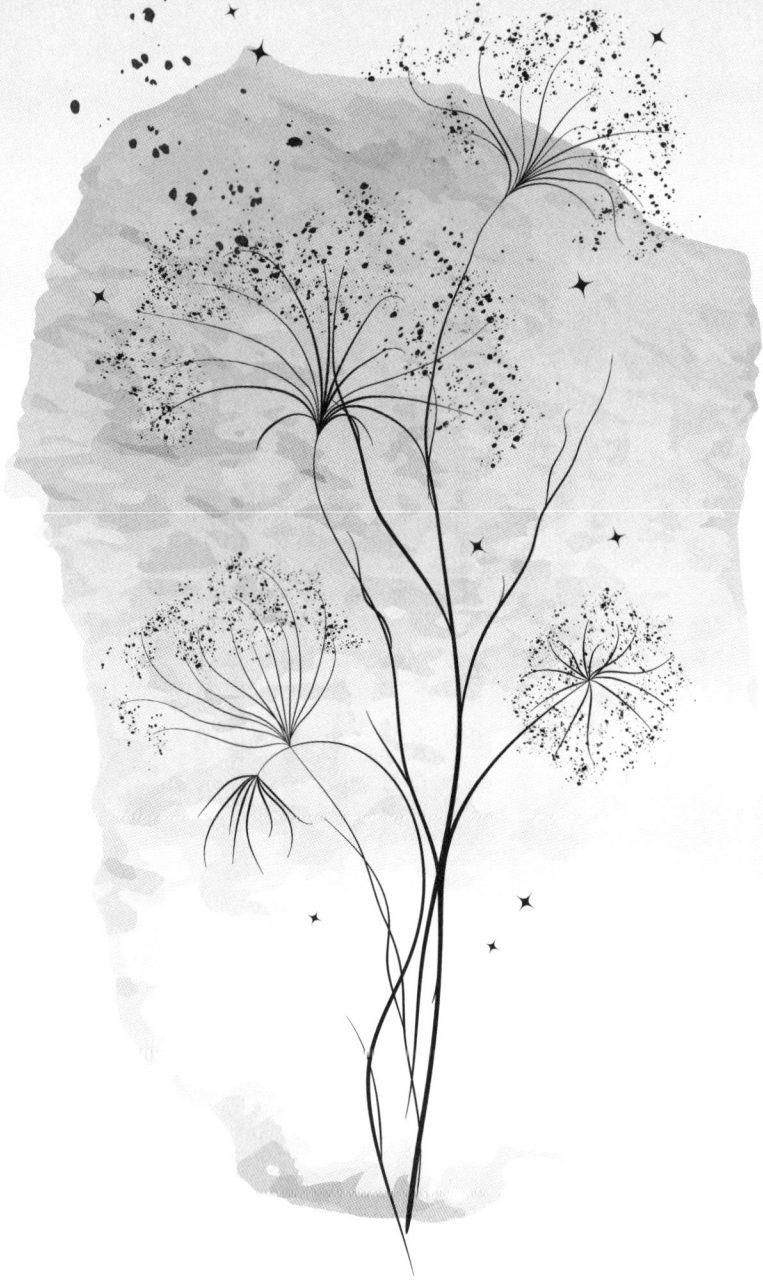

WHO IS THIS JOURNAL FOR?

Anyone who believes they are mortal. Yes, that's you! Whether you are in your golden years or just embarking on your adult life, this journal will take you by the hand and guide you down a path toward exploring your own mortality.

HOW TO USE THIS JOURNAL

This journal is divided into five sections. Each section builds on the previous one, so it's best to complete them sequentially—at your own pace. It's fine to skip a prompt and return to it later but try not to skip more than two prompts in a row.

While working through this journal, unexpected thoughts and feelings might come up for you. Try to be honest. Allow yourself to be vulnerable. Keep that tissue box nearby.

I have found that it's easy to get overly cerebral with this topic. For that reason, it can be helpful to bring your attention back to the present. The activities at the end of each section will give you the chance to integrate what you have journaled about and engage with the material on both an intellectual and emotional level. After you finish a section, you get to check in with yourself and decide whether to move forward or if it's time for a break.

··· ✦ ···

This journal is an invitation to meditate on your impermanence. So, find a pen, draw yourself a bath, and start marinating in your own mortality.

Come on in, the water is fine.

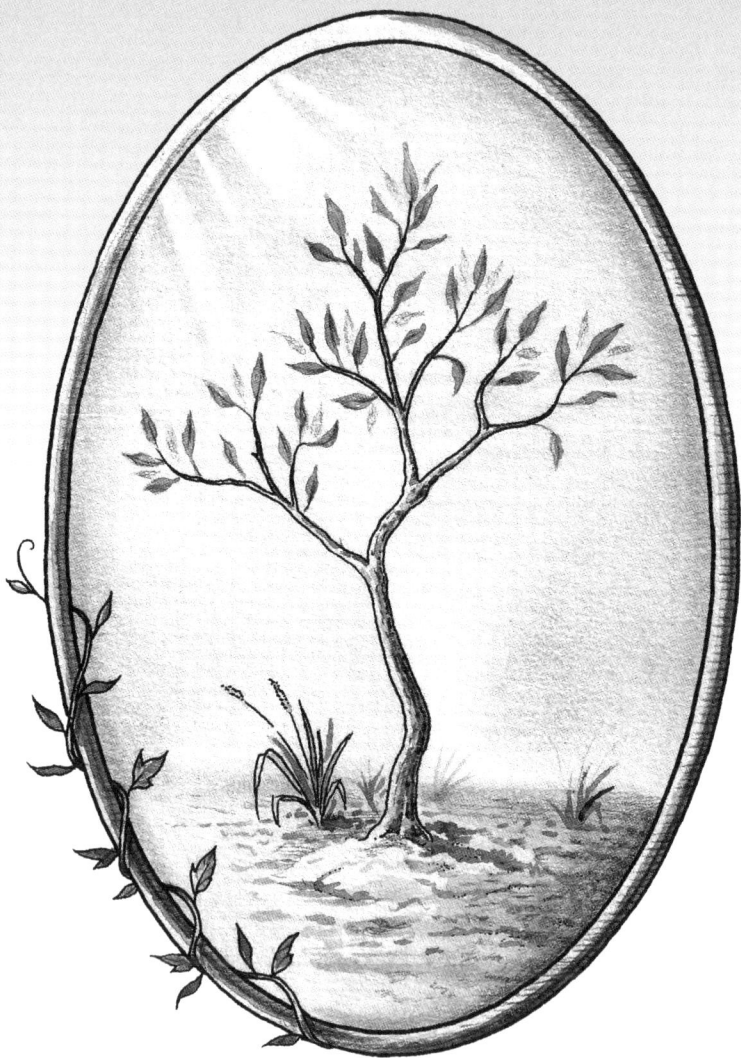

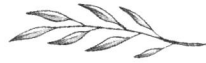

my
STARTING
POINTS

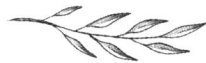

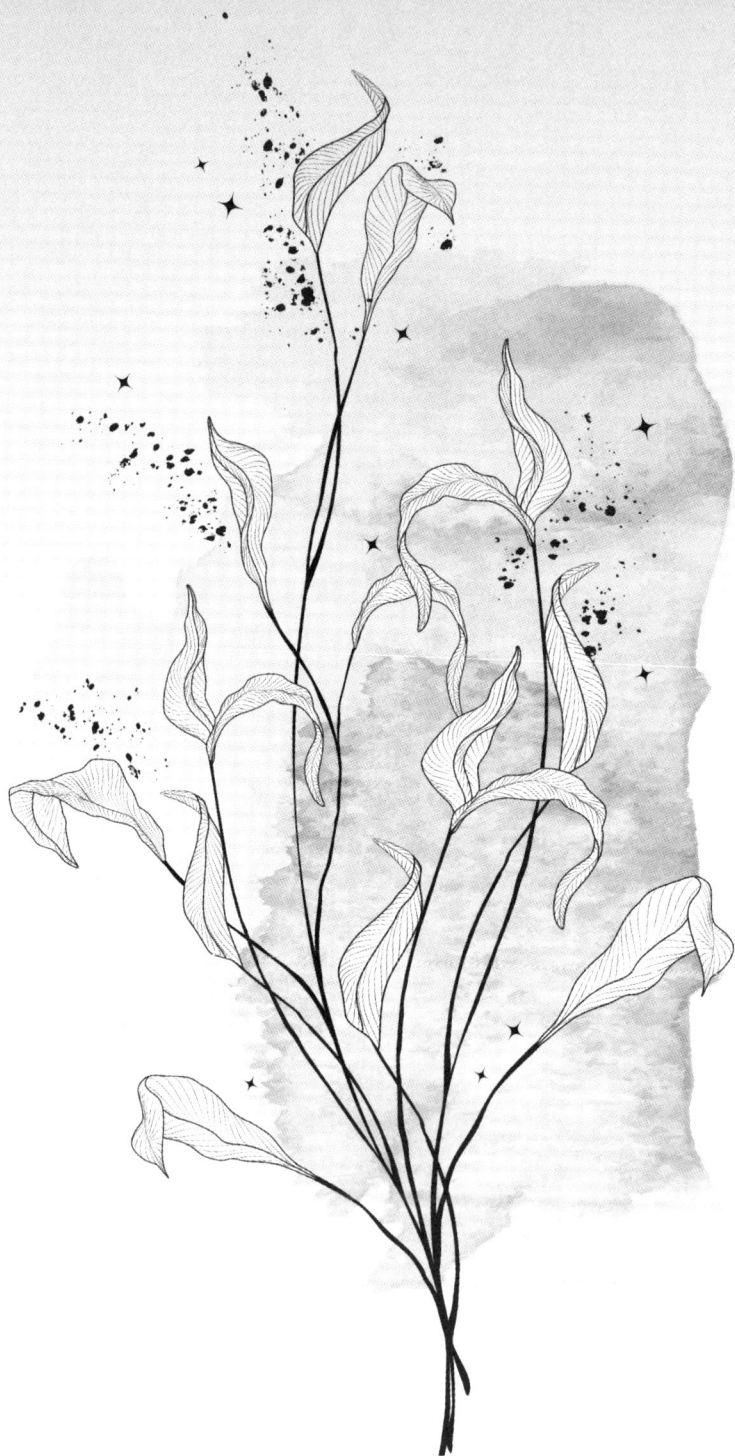

In a world that wants you to think that everything is infinite, turning toward your mortality is something of a radical act. In our modern culture, we have pushed death squarely into the shadows. For most of us, death has become nearly invisible— tucked away in nursing homes and hospitals, silenced in everyday conversation, and outsourced to funeral professionals.

It's not just that we usually don't see death up close anymore. In much of the Western world, the end of life has become so medicalized that death is often viewed as a failure, rather than an expected part of life. Think of all the hospital shows we consume on TV: the drama is always at its height when someone flatlines.

And yet, when human beings try to sidestep their mortality— when they attempt to deny death—facing its presence becomes incredibly painful. If death has become an enemy to be defeated, we will always be losing the war.

In this first section, I invite you to explore your previous exposure to death and dying.

What did you grow up believing about death as a child or young adult? Who taught you about death?

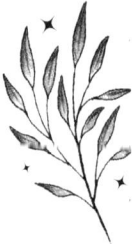

Have your views on death evolved since then? If so, how?

Who has died in your life that was close to you? How have you
processed these deaths?

Have you ever seen a dead body in real life? If so, what were the circumstances and how did it make you feel? If not, why do you think you haven't?

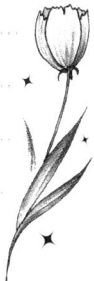

Does death play any part in your day-to-day life now?

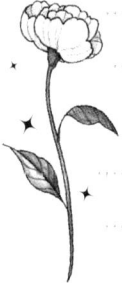

What have you observed about our cultural tendency to deny death?
Where and when have you encountered it?

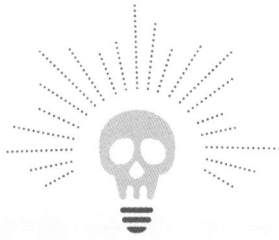

DID YOU KNOW?

In the Victorian era, people were much more familiar with many aspects of death. Back then, most people took care of their own dead, who usually died at home.

As part of their dollhouse accessories, young girls used to receive death kits to help them understand and practice proper death rituals and etiquette. These kits consisted of a doll with black mourning clothes and a coffin. Girls would hold wakes and put on funerals for their dolls—just as they were expected to do for their families when they grew up.

How do you think our views on youth and aging play into this tendency to deny death?

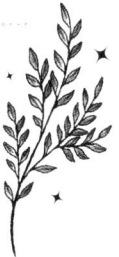

What have you observed about speaking about death? Have you tried to bring up this subject before? What do you recall about people's reactions?

What do you think is lost when we don't think or talk about death?

Are you familiar with different approaches toward human mortality, perhaps from other cultural and religious contexts?

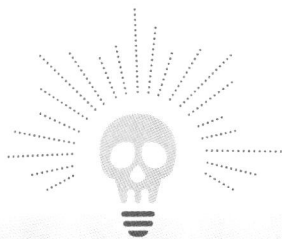

DID YOU KNOW?

In societies where people spend time preparing for the end of their lives, there's a far greater acceptance of death. For instance, among Hyolmo Buddhists in Nepal, dying is regarded as an intricate art to be studied throughout one's lifetime. The goal is to ensure a smooth passage into the next life as well as a successful rebirth.

The dying cannot accomplish such a weighty task by themselves. Relatives assist the dying person in dissolving their attachments to the world. They might place valued objects, such as money or jewelry, on the dying person's chest to satisfy any lingering yearnings for possessions in this world. When death approaches, those near and far gather at the deathbed to prevent the dying person from being held back by their longing for loved ones.

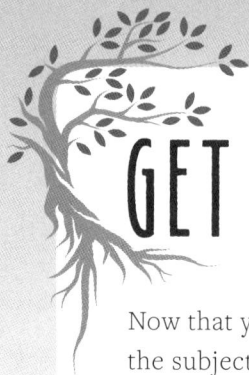

GET GROUNDED

Now that you've begun to consider your previous exposure to the subject of death, I invite you to broaden your circle and bring in community. Please pick any of the following options:

1. Initiate a **conversation** with a loved one about any aspect of death and dying. This could be a parent, sibling, or partner. Try to have it over a meal or in an otherwise relaxed setting. There's no need for a set agenda. Just try to broach the topic and see where it goes.

    OR

2. Put together or attend a more structured event for talking about death.

    Find out if there's a local chapter of a **Death Cafe**, a community gathering over tea and cake with the purpose of talking about death. There might also be a virtual option to join. More info can be found here: **deathcafe.com**.

    Alternatively, think about hosting a **Death Over Dinner**, an interactive event for families and friends to have a conversation about the end of life. For more information and detailed instructions, visit **deathoverdinner.org**.

How did that activity go? Who did you engage with? What thoughts or emotions came up for you?

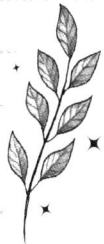

CHECKING IN ✓

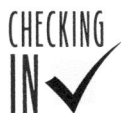

How do you feel after this initial foray into your mortality? Circle all the emotions that are rising to the surface.

Accepting	Humbled	Restless
Afraid	Intrigued	Sad
Amazed	Invigorated	Satisfied
Ambivalent	Liberated	Sentimental
Anxious	Light	Serene
Apprehensive	Melancholic	Stressed
Astonished	Nervous	Stuck
Calm	Nostalgic	Surprised
Confident	Optimistic	Tender
Content	Overwhelmed	Thankful
Curious	Pleased	Trusting
Delighted	Powerless	Pensive
Disoriented	Puzzled	Uncertain
Empowered	Rattled	Uneasy
Fascinated	Relaxed	Validated
Glum	Relieved	Vulnerable
Hopeful	Remorseful	Worried

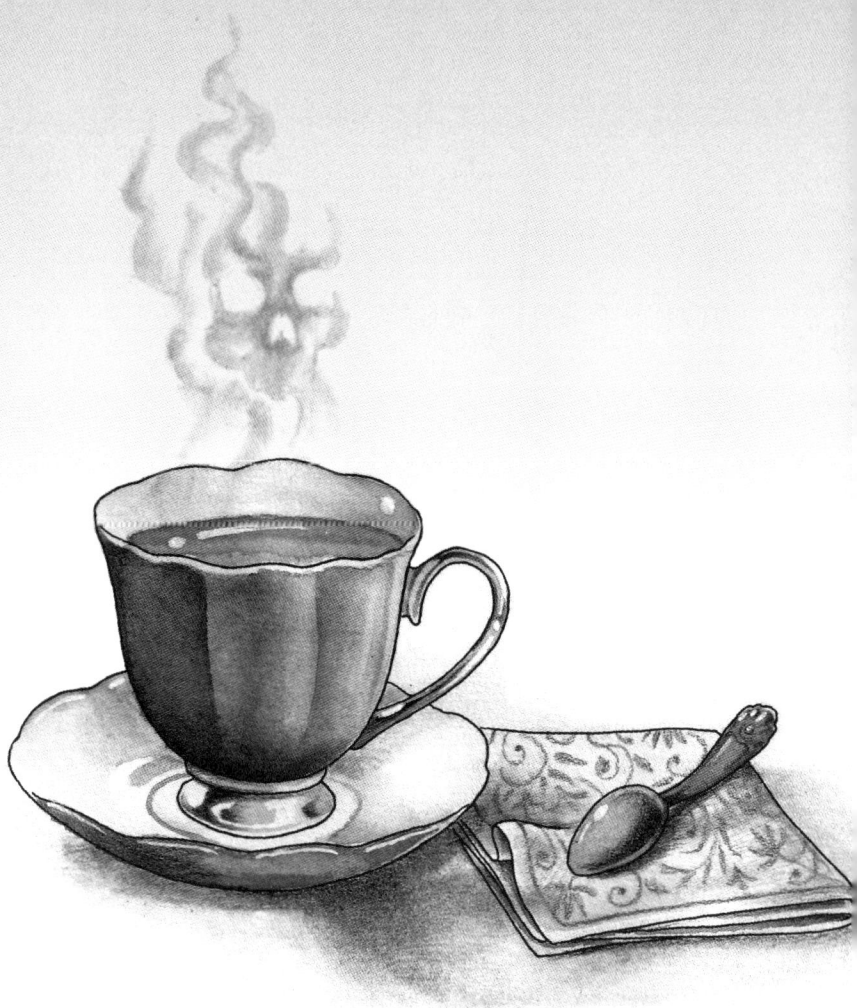

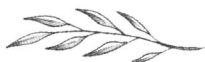

MY
FEARS

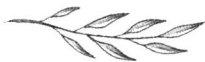

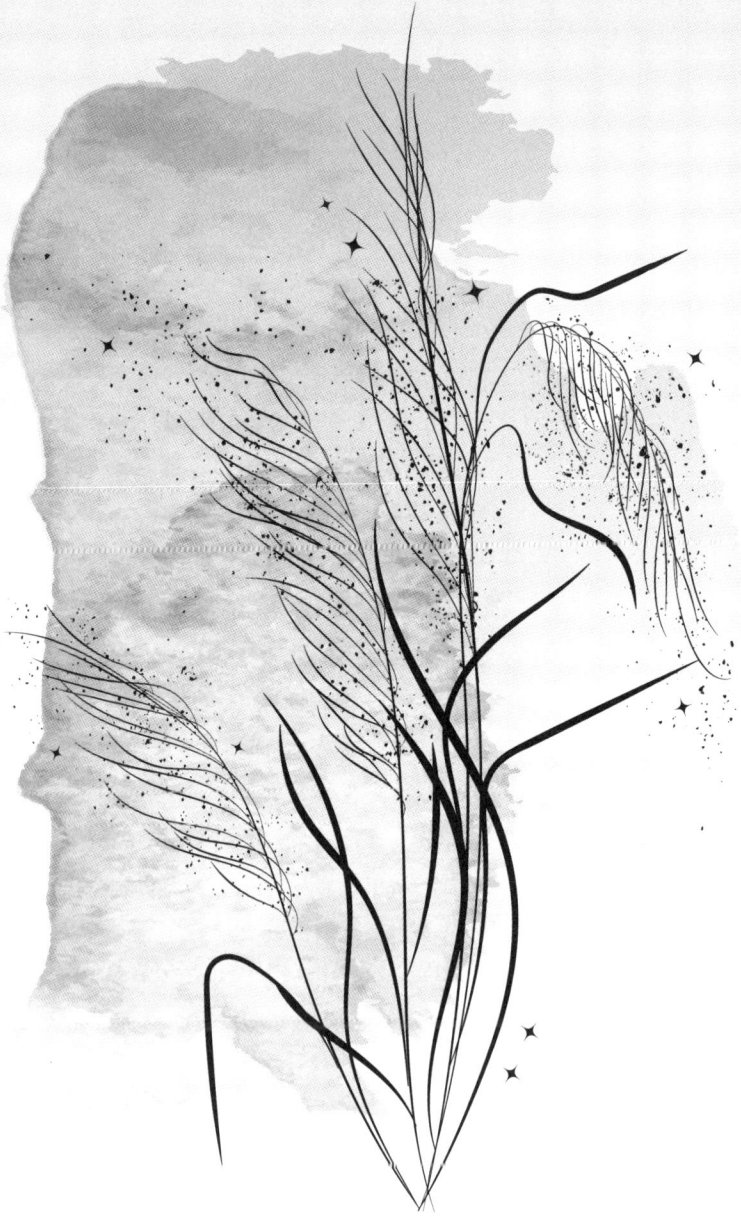

Some psychologists believe that human beings have an innate fear of death. Our terror of death, they suggest, is part of a critical instinct of self-preservation. Most of the time, we repress this fear because dwelling on it would paralyze us.

Others have argued that our fear of death is entirely learned—that our upbringing and social environment teach us to be afraid of death. They point to the fact that young children seem to have no intrinsic fear of death.

Whatever the case, dreading death diminishes our ability to enjoy the transient gift that is life.

In this second section, I invite you to contemplate some of your fears around death and dying.

What do you fear most about death and dying?

What feelings arise when you dwell on that fear?

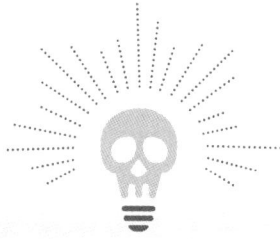

DID YOU KNOW?

Studies have shown that psilocybin, the psychedelic substance found in magic mushrooms, can substantially decrease death anxiety in patients with advanced cancer. After a single treatment, participants in one clinical trial reported feeling much less afraid and more accepting of death. They also described gaining meaningful psychological and spiritual insights for their life. Even six months after the initial dose, these effects were sustained.

If you could control one thing about your death—the time, the place, or how you die—which would you choose and why?

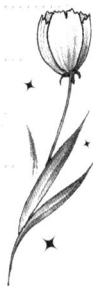

What is the closest near-death experience you had? What effects did it have on your life?

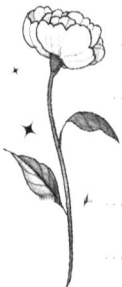

Imagine you knew precisely when you were going to die. Would you live differently? If so, how?

What deceased person would you like to have a conversation with? What would you want to know?

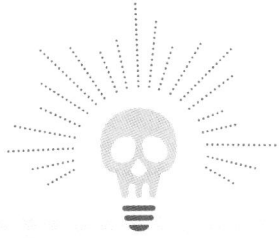

DID YOU KNOW?

A hydra is a freshwater polyp that scientists believe to be virtually immortal. Left to its own devices, the hydra's cells regenerate endlessly, making it impervious to death. Every twenty days, the entire organism renews itself.

Scientists have used the famed creature's cells in studies on aging and healing, but they still aren't completely sure what causes the hydra's infinite youthfulness.

Imagine for a second that you could be immortal.

Here are the terms: you would not continue to age, everyone you know would also be immortal (if they choose to be), and you would not bear the physical traces of normally fatal accidents. Would you do it?

☐ Definitely—that sounds amazing.

☐ Eternal life? No, thank you.

Why?

Write a (love) note to death.

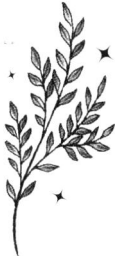

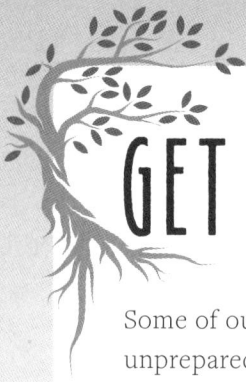

GET GROUNDED

Some of our death-related fears stem from feeling unprepared for life's final chapter. One way to prepare is to let others know about your end-of-life wishes in advance—in the event that you can no longer decide for yourself. An advance care directive (or living will) is a document that details what medical treatment—if any—you want at the end of your life and who should be the person making decisions on your behalf (your "healthcare proxy").

1. Go to **caringinfo.org** and search for "advance directives." You will find links to your state's form, along with instructions. **Fill out** an advance care directive.

    OR

2. If you've already filled out an advance care directive, **revisit** the document. Make sure it still reflects your wishes and check in with your healthcare proxy about whether they are up to date on what exactly you want to happen.

How did that activity go? What thoughts or emotions came up
for you?

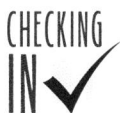

How do you feel after thinking through your fears in relationship to death? Circle all the emotions that are rising to the surface.

Accepting	Humbled	Restless
Afraid	Intrigued	Sad
Amazed	Invigorated	Satisfied
Ambivalent	Liberated	Sentimental
Anxious	Light	Serene
Apprehensive	Melancholic	Stressed
Astonished	Nervous	Stuck
Calm	Nostalgic	Surprised
Confident	Optimistic	Tender
Content	Overwhelmed	Thankful
Curious	Pleased	Trusting
Delighted	Powerless	Pensive
Disoriented	Puzzled	Uncertain
Empowered	Rattled	Uneasy
Fascinated	Relaxed	Validated
Glum	Relieved	Vulnerable
Hopeful	Remorseful	Worried

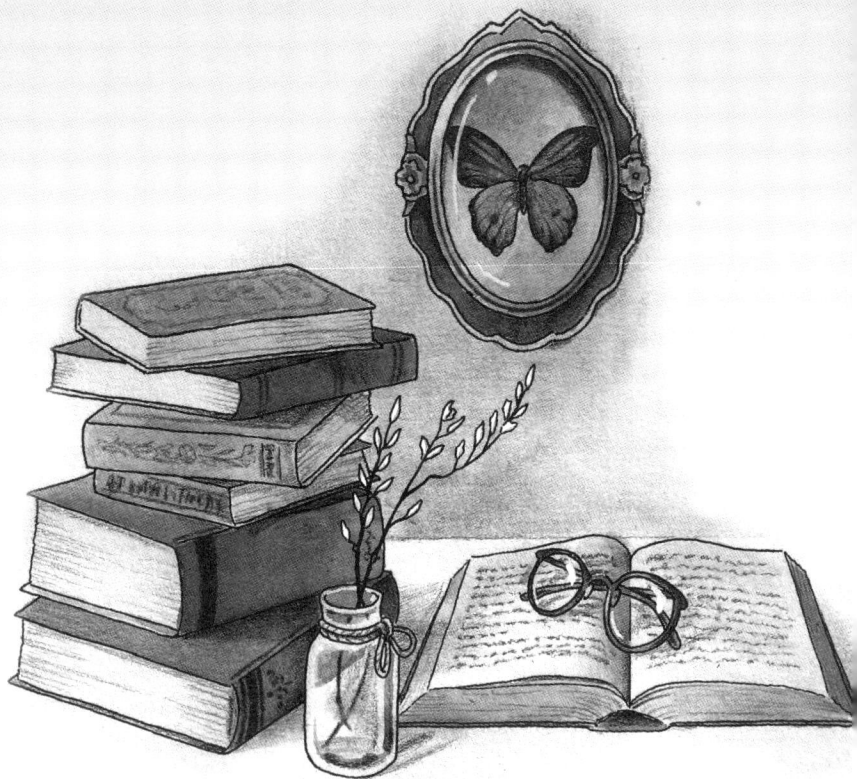

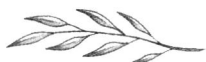

MY
LEGACY

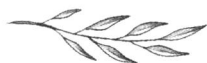

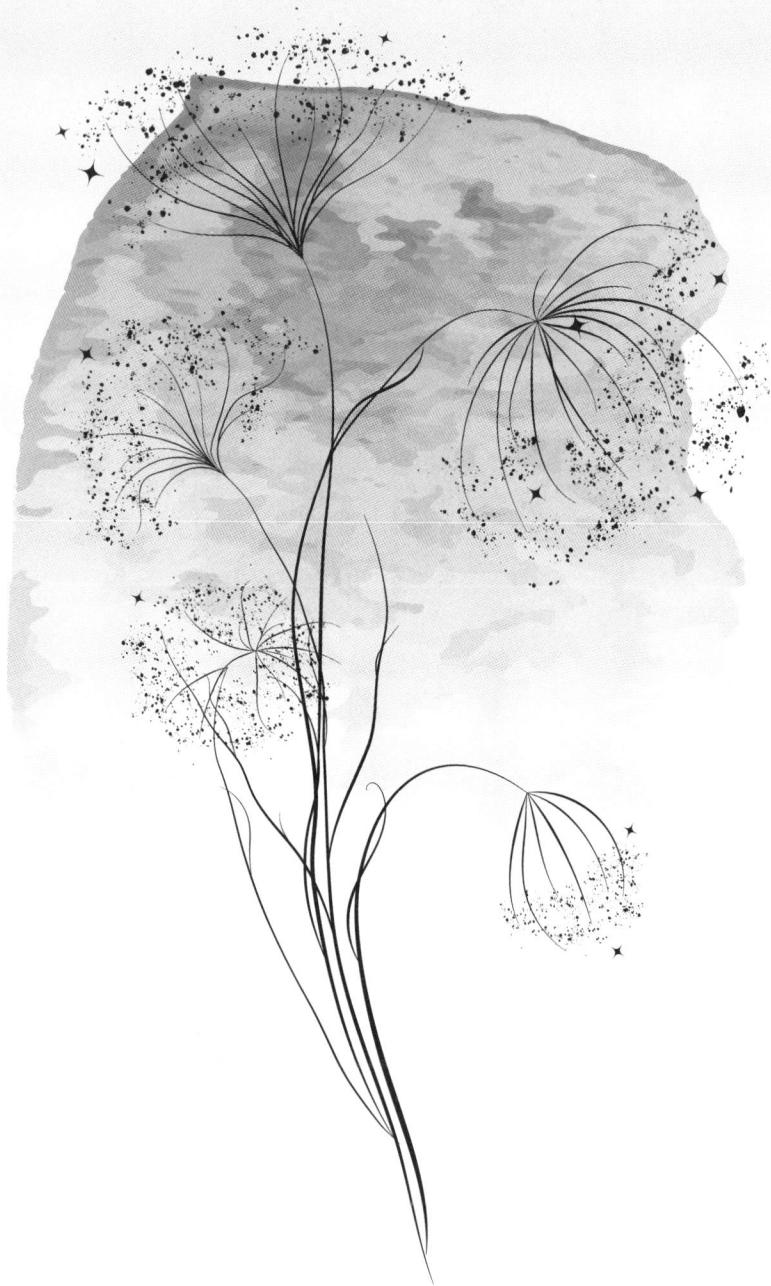

We don't often stop to assess our life and what it all means.
Especially when you are young, it can be difficult to think about your legacy. *What have I done*, you might ask, *that has been of any consequence?*

But legacy work isn't only about chronicling the past. It's about remembering who you are and where you came from; it's a return to your authentic self. Which challenges have you already overcome? How might you use these experiences to meet new challenges in the future?

In this third section, I invite you to recall the resilience, competencies, and strengths you have shown in the past to equip you for what lies ahead—in life as in death. Ask yourself one big question: What do I want to leave behind?

Looking at your life right now, how would you describe your guiding principles? What are your core values?

How have you lived these values? Identify some concrete examples.

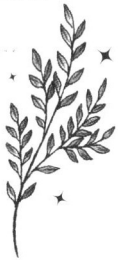

What is one difficult experience you are grateful you had?

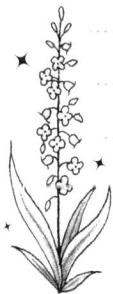

What was the biggest risk you ever took? What was at stake, and what did you learn from it?

If you could relive one moment in your life, which would it be?
Would you change it or keep it the same?

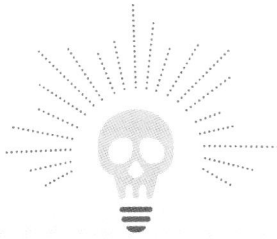

DID YOU KNOW?

Have you ever considered that you could be carrying the legacy of another within your body?

When a person is pregnant, the cells of the developing fetus become embedded in their own body. During gestation, fetal cells migrate through the placenta and integrate into the parent's tissue, where they can remain for decades. Scientists have discovered fetal cells living in their parent's skin, lungs, heart, and brain even after the parent dies.

Strange as it may sound, many of us bear remnants of other people inside us.

What is something that aging has taught you about life? (Even if you are still young, there are likely life lessons you've learned since emerging from your teenage years.)

What is the best piece of advice you ever received?

If you could share one piece of advice with the next generation, what would it be?

Who are the most significant mentors in your life? Jot down a few things they taught you.

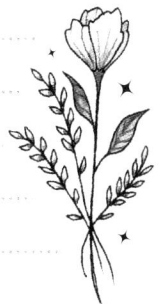

What is the most important thing you want people to remember about you?

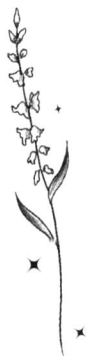

....

....

....

....

....

....

....

....

....

....

....

....

....

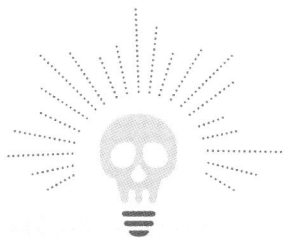

DID YOU KNOW?

Over the past decade, growing numbers of South Koreans of all ages have sought out "mock funerals"—community events that stage participants' deaths. Mock funerals take place in large softly lit halls filled with individual wooden coffins. Attendees have their "final" photograph taken and framed, don a ceremonial robe, write their last testament, and lie down inside a coffin as an attendant closes the lid. They stay motionless for ten minutes.

Participants say that undergoing a dry run for their own deaths helped them discover a new approach to life and realize that happiness resides in the present.

Imagine that you booked a South Korean mock funeral. You climb into the coffin, the properly ventilated lid closes, and it's just you and your thoughts. What do you feel proudest of? Don't be modest. Think of all the ways—big and small—you have touched other people's lives (interpersonally, professionally, athletically, creatively, and through your mere existence).

You are still in that coffin. What do you regret?

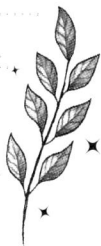

What did you never get a chance to say? To whom?

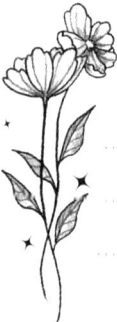

What do you want your future legacy to be? What enduring dreams and ambitions do you have?

What are five things you want to do before you die?

What are five more things?

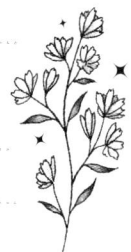

Which of these things can you get started on **right now**?

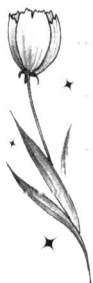

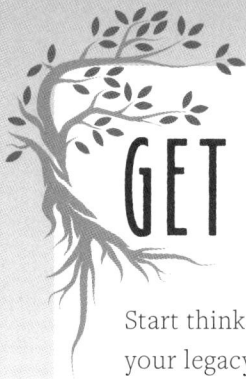

GET GROUNDED

Start thinking of small but concrete ways of **preserving** your legacy. Here are some ideas:

1. Write down your best recipes.

2. Record that song you've been working on.

3. Make a two-minute video for a loved one.

4. Write a letter to someone and keep it in a drawer.

5. Plant something in the ground.

6. Start a new photo album.

Whatever it is, decide on a small project you can complete right now.

How did that activity go? What thoughts and emotions came up for you as you completed it?

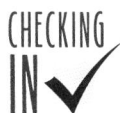

How do you feel after thinking about what you will leave behind and what you still want to do? Circle all the emotions that are rising to the surface.

Afraid	Intrigued	Sad
Amazed	Invigorated	Satisfied
Ambivalent	Liberated	Sentimental
Anxious	Light	Serene
Apprehensive	Melancholic	Stressed
Astonished	Nervous	Stuck
Calm	Nostalgic	Surprised
Confident	Optimistic	Tender
Content	Overwhelmed	Thankful
Curious	Pleased	Trusting
Delighted	Powerless	Pensive
Disoriented	Puzzled	Uncertain
Empowered	Rattled	Uneasy
Fascinated	Relaxed	Validated
Glum	Relieved	Vulnerable
Hopeful	Remorseful	Worried
Humbled	Restless	

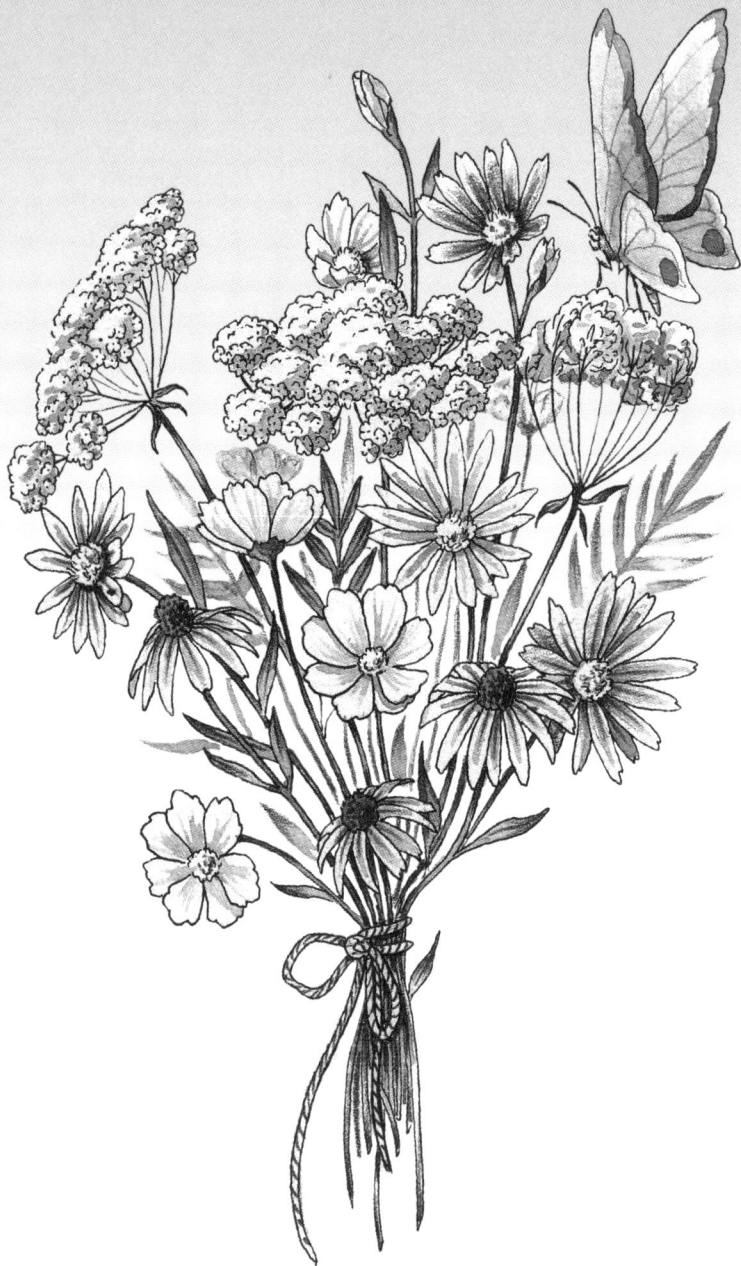

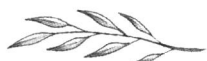

MY
DEATH

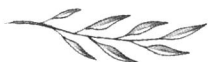

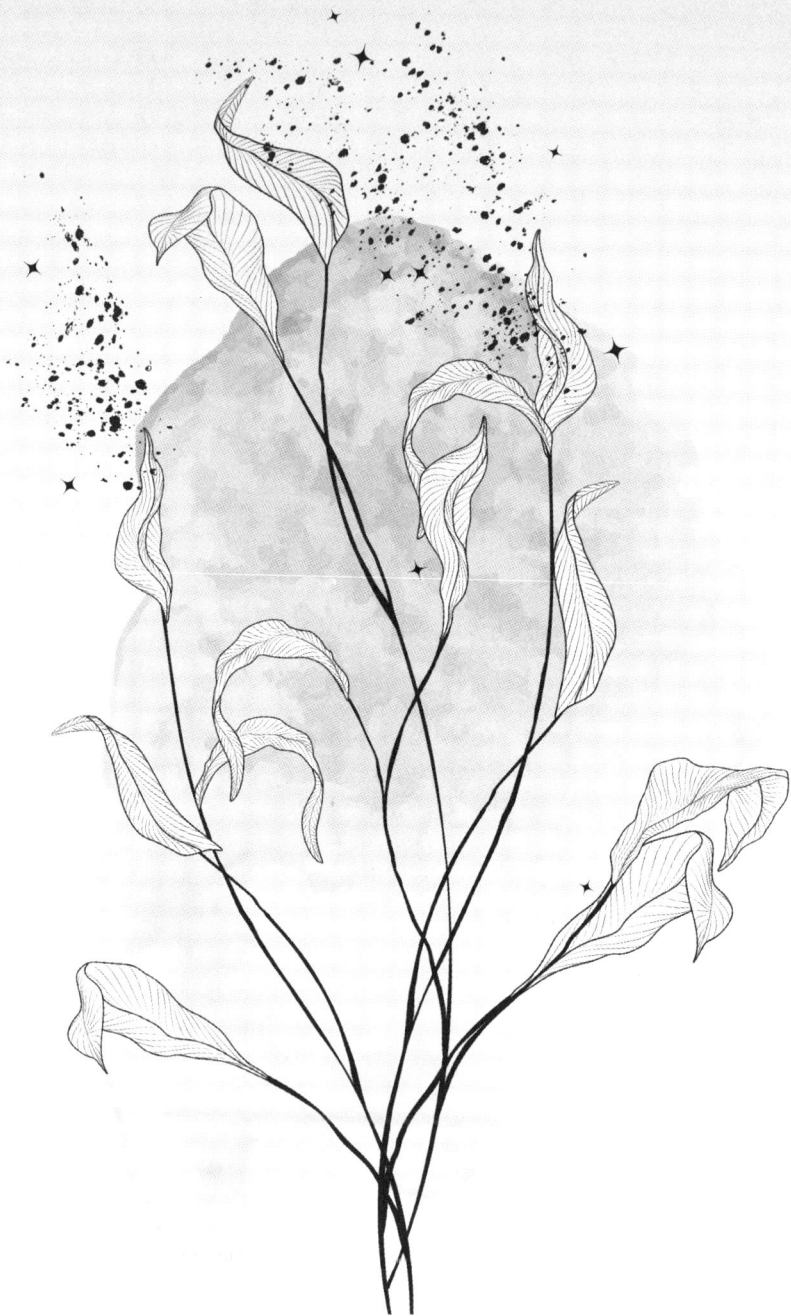

Nice work! You've made it over halfway through your mortality journal. I hope you feel a sense of accomplishment.

This fourth section will require all your focus: it centers on your own death. But don't worry, you have been here before. If you have ever been to a yoga class, you have likely spent at least part of your session in corpse pose, or Shavasana. And even if you don't practice yoga, the work you have put into this journal so far has more than equipped you to tackle this section.

So, take a deep breath and dive in with me.

What does "dying well" mean to you? What constitutes a "good death" in your eyes? Think about all the potential elements—the mental and physical state of the dying person, their stage in life, and the manner and circumstances of their death.

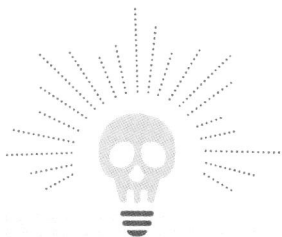

DID YOU KNOW?

Originally, the word *euthanasia*—derived from the Greek words *eu* (*good* or *well*) and *thanatos* (*death*)— meant *a good death*. Between the late Middle Ages and the Enlightenment, a good death wasn't necessarily a painless death.

At the time, popular manuals on the art of dying, *Ars moriendi*, coached readers on how to comport themselves on their deathbeds to guarantee their salvation. Priests who were called to the beds of the dying used the manuals to help prepare the pious for their deaths. Back then, dying well meant fighting earthly temptations by embodying virtues such as faith, patience, and humility.

It was only once physicians replaced clergy at the deathbed in the nineteenth century that the term *euthanasia* came to signify a painless death. At the end of that century, *euthanasia* took on the meaning it still has today: the use of lethal medications at the hands of a clinician to bring about a quick and painless death.

What would your dream death look like? Where are you? Who is there? What are you wearing? How does it all unfold?

What's your ideal state of mind on your deathbed?

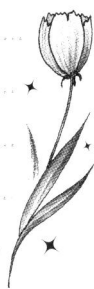

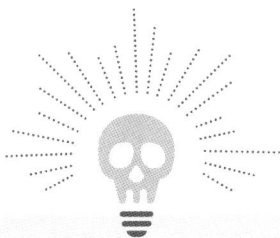

DID YOU KNOW?

In many ways, dying is a continuous exercise in letting go. As the dying person dissolves their attachments to the world, their loved ones work on releasing them emotionally. Rituals can play a key role in this process. They offer direction and meaning to an otherwise destabilizing experience—a way to honor a dying person in the very process of letting them go.

Death doulas can help with these transitions. They provide important emotional, physical, and spiritual comfort and assist with the many logistic aspects of dying. Some of them are versed in the power of ritual and can help design a guided ceremony for the person who is dying.

What do you imagine would help you let go and surrender when it's time for you to die? To help answer this question, practice by lying down and imagine sinking into the ground beneath you.

What do you imagine would help your loved ones release you? Is there anything you could do to help them let go?

Is there a religious or spiritual dimension that's important to you when you think about your death?

What do you think happens to you after you die?

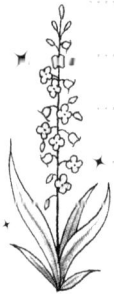

Since you started journaling, what new revelations have you had about death?

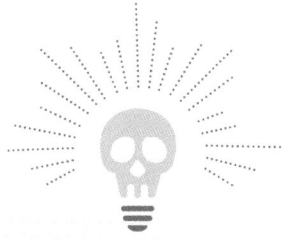

DID YOU KNOW?

During my time studying medical aid in dying, I got to know many people who had made peace with death. Their physical and emotional suffering had melted away any desire to live, and they found great solace in being able to hasten their own death. Most had accepted the hard truth of their mortality and looked to their own passing with a sense of completion.

Many of us associate this moment with the word *terminal*. But in my experience, these endings were also a form of liberation—a path clearing toward an unknown horizon.

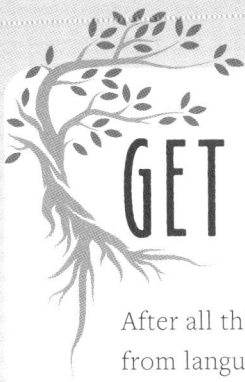

GET GROUNDED

After all this cerebral work, I invite you to release yourself from language and drop back into your body.

Light a **candle**, make yourself a cup of **tea**, and pick several **colors** that resonate with you. As you color in this mandala, meditate on what it might mean to live—from this moment on—with the full awareness of your mortality. Knowing all that you know now, how could you live with intention and purpose in the time you have remaining?

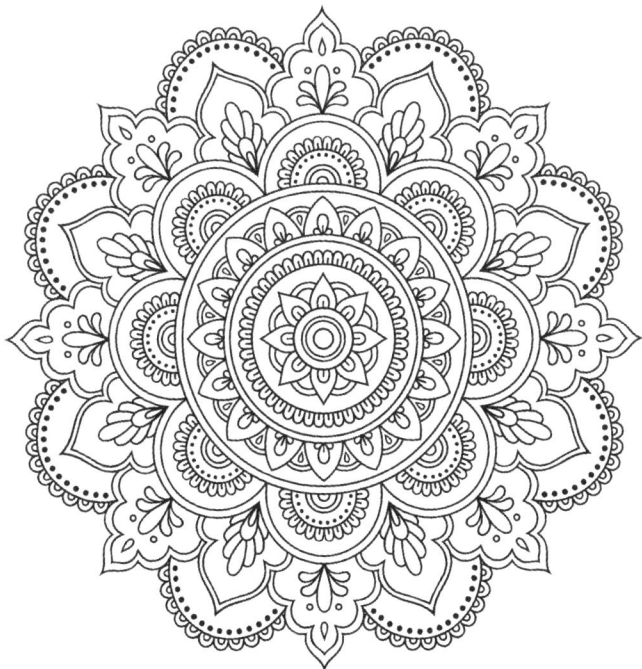

How did that coloring exercise go? What thoughts and emotions came up for you?

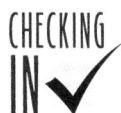

How do you feel after contemplating your own death? Circle all the emotions that are rising to the surface.

Afraid	Intrigued	Sad
Amazed	Invigorated	Satisfied
Ambivalent	Liberated	Sentimental
Anxious	Light	Serene
Apprehensive	Melancholic	Stressed
Astonished	Nervous	Stuck
Calm	Nostalgic	Surprised
Confident	Optimistic	Tender
Content	Overwhelmed	Thankful
Curious	Pleased	Trusting
Delighted	Powerless	Pensive
Disoriented	Puzzled	Uncertain
Empowered	Rattled	Uneasy
Fascinated	Relaxed	Validated
Glum	Relieved	Vulnerable
Hopeful	Remorseful	Worried
Humbled	Restless	

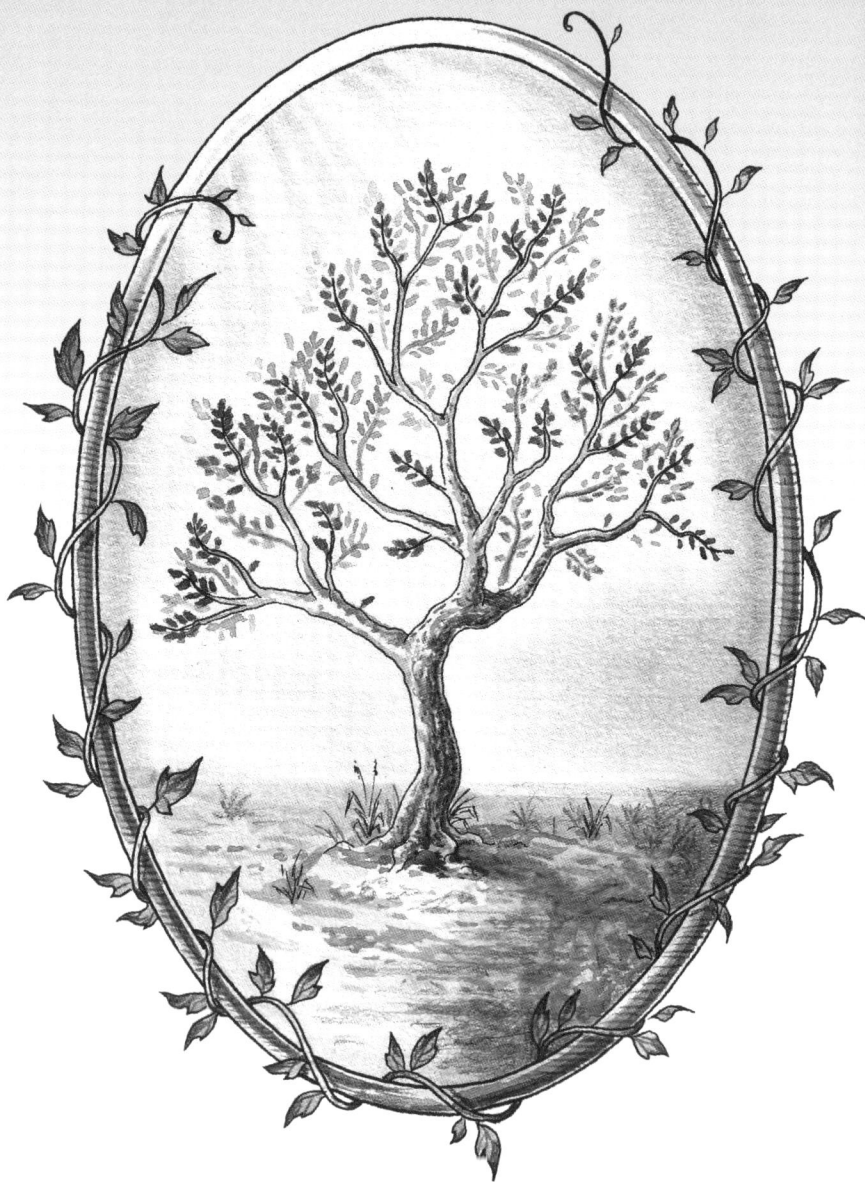

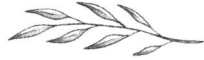

MY
MEMORIAL

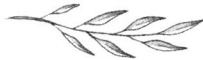

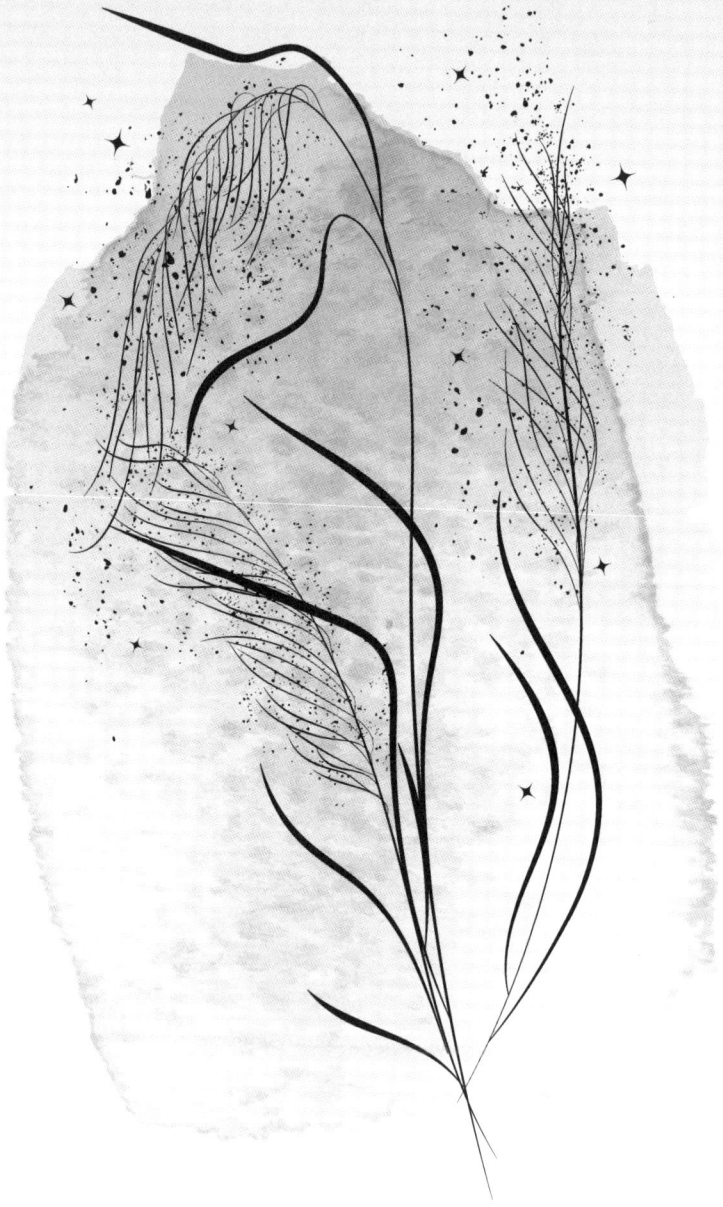

Nowadays, there are lots of ways to be memorialized. Depending on where you live, you can opt for a traditional burial, a green burial, cremation, or aquamation (also known as *water* or *flameless cremation*). Some states now have provisions for human composting, and in Colorado you can dispose of your body on an open-air funeral pyre. You can choose to donate your body to science, or you can turn your ashes into a diamond or press them into a vinyl record.

Those who feel uncomfortable with the finality of death have options too. Scientists are studying ways to "download" a person's brain so they can continue to live virtually after death. Then there's cryonics, the practice of freezing bodies or body parts in the hope that future scientists will thaw them and bring them back to life.

Or perhaps you feel satisfied with your name on a park bench, or leaving no trace at all.

In this final section, I invite you to think about how you would like to be memorialized.

What do you want to happen with your body after you die? What appeals to you about this option?

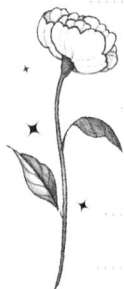

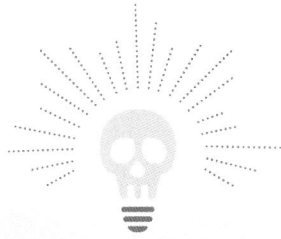

DID YOU KNOW?

Some societies grieve and recover from the loss of a loved one by erasing all traces of their existence. Among the indigenous people of the Wari' in Brazil, the grieving process long entailed destroying the deceased's property and crops, rerouting the forest paths that led to their home, and avoiding saying their name. Until the 1960s, in-laws of the deceased would also consume parts of the body to help make the corpse disappear—widely regarded as a compassionate and honorable thing to do.

Severing all relationships to the deceased and eradicating any reminders of them helped the bereaved accept their loss and move on with their lives.

Do you prefer to leave a trace of yourself or no trace at all?

In what other ways would you like to be memorialized?

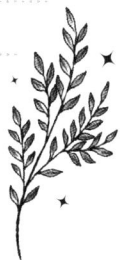

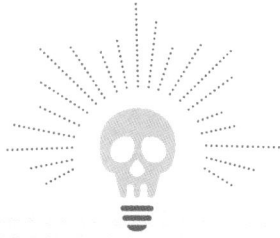

DID YOU KNOW?

The last two decades have seen a resurgence in natural home death care. Instead of relinquishing the deceased's body to mortuary staff right away, families are increasingly opting to perform the postmortem bodily care themselves. With the body resting on packs of ice, families wash and anoint the deceased with special oils, clean and style their hair, and dress them in their chosen outfit. They might invite relatives and friends to hold vigil until it's time for the funeral.

Many report feeling intensely grateful for the ability to provide this final care and for the extra time spent with their loved one.

How do you feel about the idea of having your body washed and cared for by your loved ones?

What songs, poems, or readings would you like recited at your memorial service?

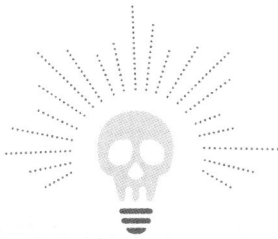

DID YOU KNOW?

Swedish death cleaning describes the practice of getting your home in order and organizing your belongings in preparation for your passing. It can be done at any stage of life and entails thoughtfully paring down your possessions to what you truly need.

Decluttering is said to benefit your loves ones after you are gone but can also help you live a more minimalist, purposeful life.

What would you like to happen with your worldly possessions after you die? Are there any belongings you feel particularly attached to? If so, why?

If you had to come up with a tongue-in-cheek inscription for your urn or gravestone, what would it be? Write or draw it.

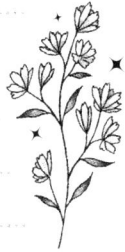

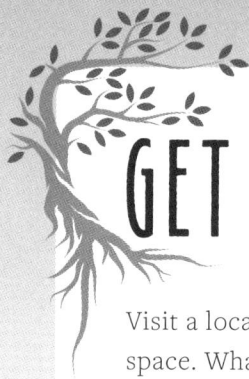

GET GROUNDED

Visit a local **cemetery** and spend some time taking in the space. What strikes you about the layout? How does this space make you feel? What information can you glean from the markers and gravestones?

1. Jot down any thoughts and observations here.

   OR

2. If you are unable to visit a cemetery, what do you **recall** about previous visits?

How did the visit to the cemetery go? What thoughts and emotions came up for you?

CHECKING IN ✓

How do you feel after pondering the ways you would like to be memorialized? Circle all the emotions that are rising to the surface.

Accepting	Humbled	Restless
Afraid	Intrigued	Sad
Amazed	Invigorated	Satisfied
Ambivalent	Liberated	Sentimental
Anxious	Light	Serene
Apprehensive	Melancholic	Stressed
Astonished	Nervous	Stuck
Calm	Nostalgic	Surprised
Confident	Optimistic	Tender
Content	Overwhelmed	Thankful
Curious	Pleased	Trusting
Delighted	Powerless	Pensive
Disoriented	Puzzled	Uncertain
Empowered	Rattled	Uneasy
Fascinated	Relaxed	Validated
Glum	Relieved	Vulnerable
Hopeful	Remorseful	Worried

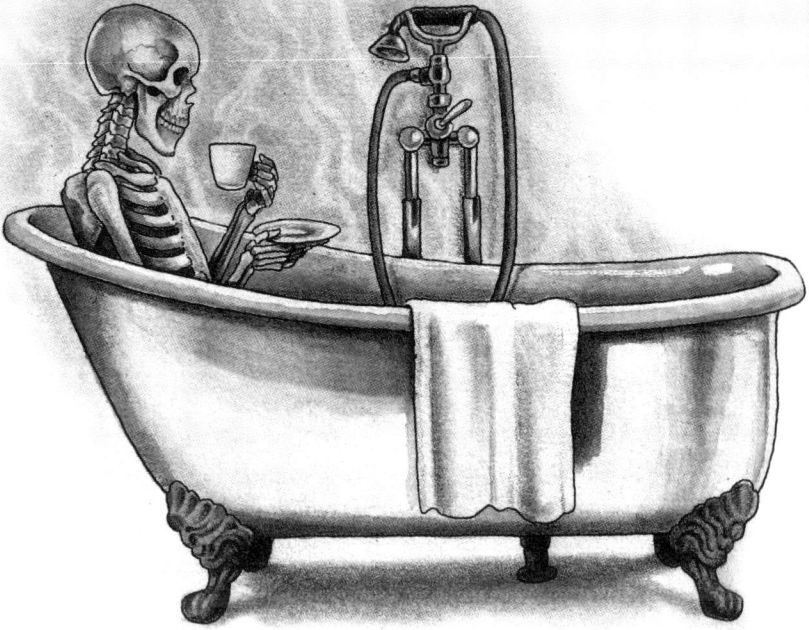

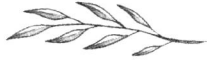

MY CLOSING THOUGHTS

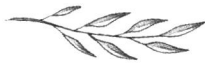

All things that seem
to die are in fact
only transformed.

Seneca, Moral Epistles

Where are you now that you've completed your mortality journal?
There are no more words to circle—just write your heart out.

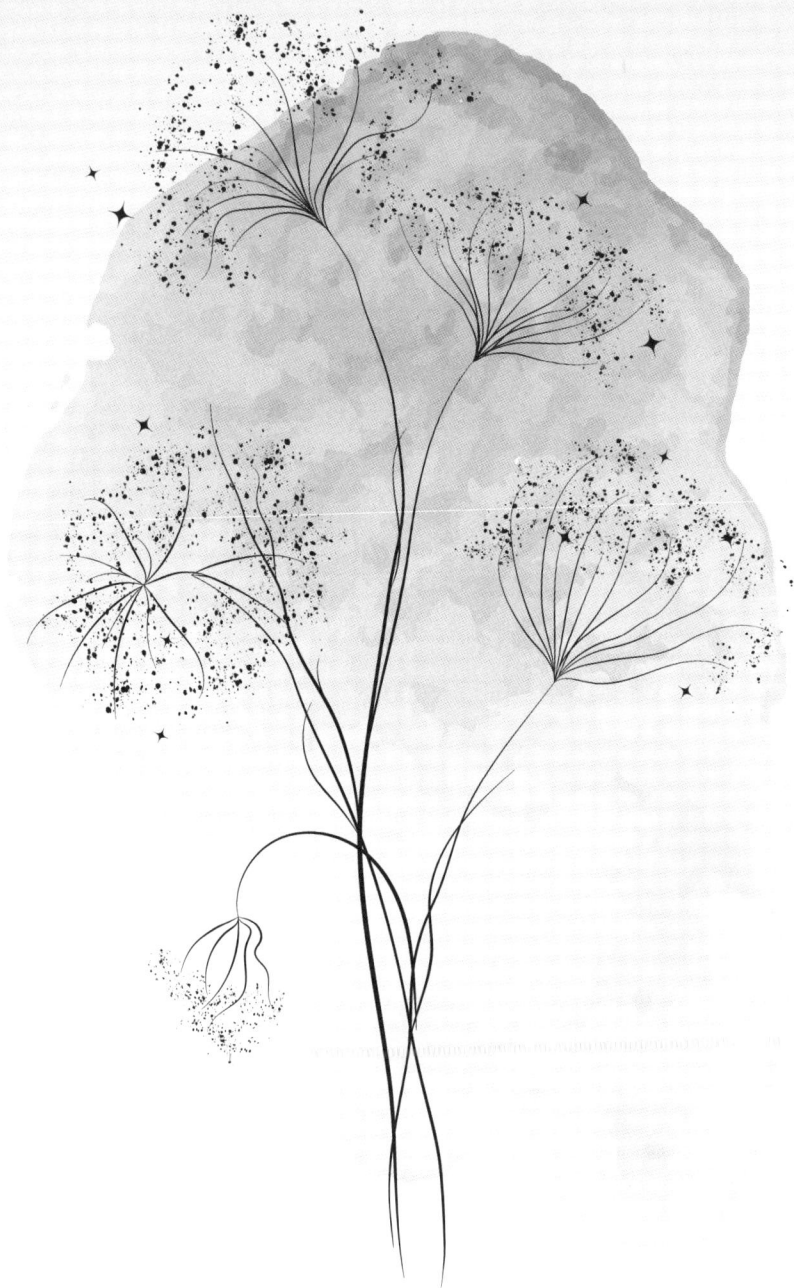

FINAL WORDS OF ENCOURAGEMENT

Dear Journaler,

Congratulations! You've just accomplished what most people never find the courage or occasion to do—you contemplated your own mortality.

Perhaps journaling about death made you reevaluate or reaffirm your priorities in life. Maybe you found something liberating—even healing—in the idea of coming face-to-face with your impermanence. Or perhaps you are still just as afraid to die as before but have gained new tools to come to terms with that fear. Wherever your process took you, I commend you for putting in the work.

I believe that finding healthy ways to think and talk about our mortality is the bedrock of a thriving society. My hope is that by encouraging these kinds of reflections in a person's life, we can regain our lost societal knowledge of death and enhance our experience of daily life.

By completing this journal, you've also taken the first step to shifting a much broader cultural conversation. I am so excited about where else this journey will take you.

Thank you for being here with me.

Anita

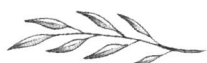

LATER
ON

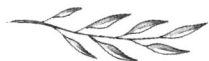

A journal doesn't have to be a snapshot of one moment in time; it can also be a living document. You might like to revisit and amend these pages a few months or years from now.

Feel free to use this space to write down any new thoughts you've had about death or any new experiences that have shifted your views on this subject.

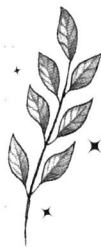

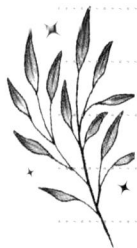

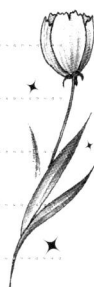

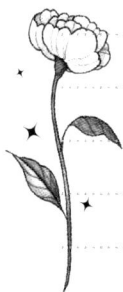

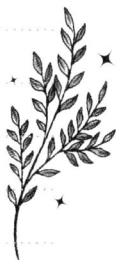

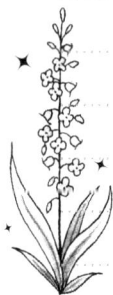

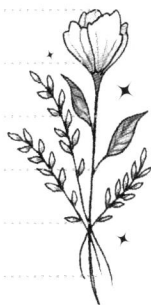

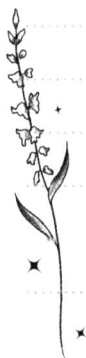

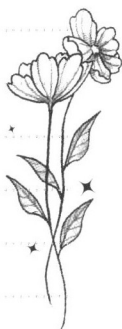

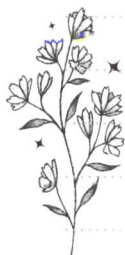

ABOUT THE AUTHOR

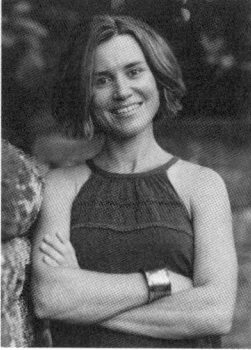

Anita Hannig is an applied anthropologist whose work explores the cultural dimensions of medicine. In recent years, Anita has emerged as a leading voice on death literacy in America, giving interviews for the *Washington Post*, *USA Today*, and the *Boston Globe*. She is the author of the critically acclaimed book *The Day I Die: The Untold Story of Assisted Dying in America*. Her writing has also appeared in *Cognoscenti*, the *Seattle Times*, and *Undark Magazine*, among other places. In her free time, Anita enjoys trail running and backpacking in the great outdoors, pursuits that sporadically bring her back in touch with her own mortality.